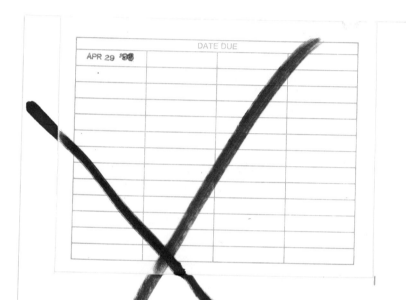

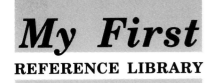

My First
REFERENCE LIBRARY

The Story of
MEDICINE

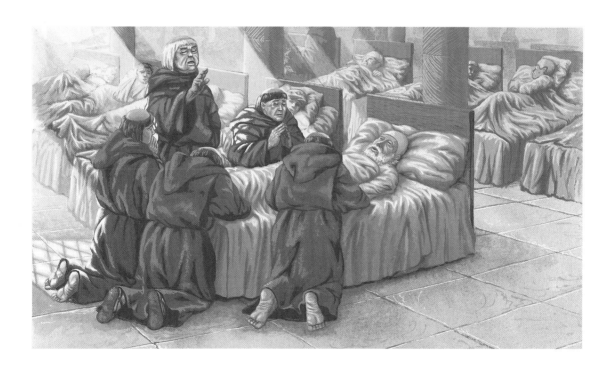

Adapted from Steve Parker's *The History of Medicine*

BARBARA BEHM

Gareth Stevens Children's Books
MILWAUKEE

For a free color catalog describing Gareth Stevens' list of high-quality children's books, call 1-800-341-3569 (USA) or 1-800-461-9120 (Canada).

Library of Congress Cataloging-in-Publication Data

Behm, Barbara, 1952-
   The story of medicine / Barbara Behm ; [illustrated by James Field, Borin van Loon, and Eugene Fleury]. — North American ed.
      p.   cm. — (My first reference library)
   Includes index.
   Summary: Examines the practice of medicine from ancient times to the present and describes its current status regarding technological advances and differing levels of expertise in different parts of the world.
   ISBN 0-8368-0049-4
   1. Medicine—History—Juvenile literature. [1. Medicine—History.] I. Field, James, ill. II. Van Loon, Borin, 1951- ill. III. Fleury, Eugene, ill. IV. Title. V. Series.
R133.5.B44   1991
610'.9—dc20   91-11739

North American edition first published in 1992 by
Gareth Stevens Children's Books
1555 North RiverCenter Drive, Suite 201
Milwaukee, Wisconsin 53212, USA

Photographic credits: Ann Ronan Picture Library 13 (left), 22 (left), 27 (top); Bibliothèque Nationale 16; Bodleian Library 11 (left); Bridgeman Art Library 4 (center); J. Allan Cash 32; Mark Edwards 50 (top); ET Archive 5, 43 (left); Format Photographers 50 (bottom); Giraudon 25 (bottom); Sally and Richard Greenhill 7 (right), 38, 57; Hulton Picture Company 30 (left), 33 (right); Hutchinson Library 47, 48, 51, 52, 53, 54 (right), 56, 58 (left), 59; Imperial War Museum 33 (left); The Independent 58 (right); John Watney Photo Library 19 (top), 27 (bottom), 30 (bottom), 39 (right), 44 (inset), 45; Magnum 4 (left), 35 (right), 42, 43 (right); Mansell Collection 13 (center), 31; Mary Evans Picture Library 13 (bottom), 36 (left); Massachusetts General Hospital 34; Master and Fellows of Trinity College, Cambridge 19 (center); National Portrait Gallery 25 (top); Österreichische National Bibliothek 17; Peter Newark's Western Americana 54 (left); Popperfoto 7 (left), 35 (top); Queen Mary's Hospital, Roehampton 44 (left); Robert Harding Picture Library 49; Ronald Sheridan's Picture Library 12, 14; Science Museum 10, 11 (right); Science Photo Library 32, 37, 39 (left), 40, 41, 43 (top), 44 (bottom); Wellcome Institute 8, 21, 22 (right); Werner Forman Archive 55; Windsor Castle, Royal Library © 1990 Her Majesty the Queen 20; ZEFA 4, 9

Illustrated by James Field, Borin van Loon, and Eugene Fleury
Cover illustration © Regis Lefebure/Third Coast

Series editors: Neil Champion and Rita Reitci
Research editor: Jennifer Thelen
Educational consultant: Dr. Alistair Ross
Designed by: Groom and Pickerill
Cover design: Beth Karpfinger
Picture research: Ann Usborne
Specialist consultant: Caroline Richmond

Printed in the United States of America

1 2 3 4 5 6 7 8 9 9 97 96 95 94 93 92

Contents

1: HEALTH AND MEDICINE

What Is Good Health?

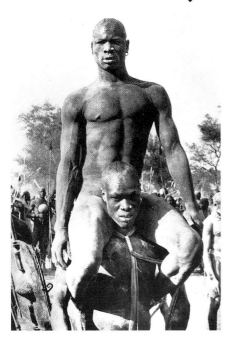

Nuba wrestlers from Africa, some of the most physically fit people in the world. ▼

Right: In the time of Queen Elizabeth I, being pale was attractive. Far right: Today, we think a suntan looks healthy. But the Sun's rays can also be harmful. ▶

Health

Most people have good health most of the time. Good health is more than just not being sick. Good health means both a healthy mind and a healthy body. People who eat a balanced diet and get plenty of exercise can fight disease better.

Illness

There are many things that can go wrong with the human body.

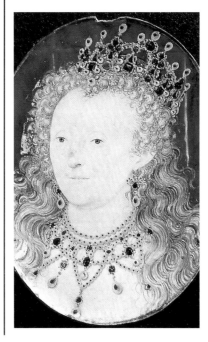

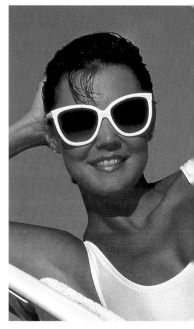

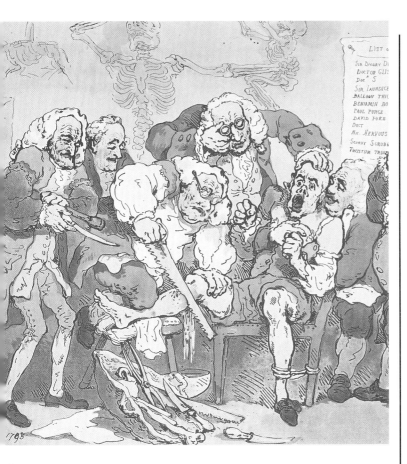

◀ This 1783 drawing shows what a terrible experience an amputation once was for the person having the operation.

People can get a disease, like measles. They can break a leg, or get an earache. When these happen, people get medical care.

Medicine

Doctors and other health workers such as chiropractors, nurses, therapists, and dentists provide medical care. They find out what is wrong with us and try to make us better. They treat us with medicine, operations, nursing, and in many other ways.

Did You Know?

A few hundred years ago, in many countries, people with mental illnesses were called "mad." There were no treatments then, so they were just locked away. This still happens today in some countries.

WHO's Health

WHO, the World Health Organization, wants the world's people to have good health. Some of WHO's work includes:

• controlling diseases, like malaria and tuberculosis

• training doctors and nurses and helping build more hospitals

• helping victims of natural disasters, like earthquakes and famine

• helping countries decide about medical care for their people.

Staying Healthy

Staying healthy means keeping in good physical condition, eating the right foods, and not getting overweight. Staying healthy means not smoking and not drinking alcohol. Staying healthy means promptly taking care of any symptoms of illness.

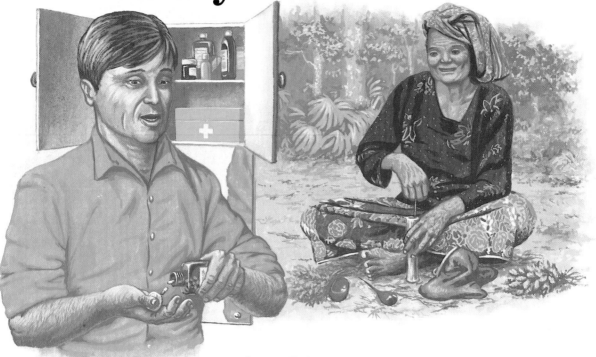

▲ Two different ways to take medicine. Above: In North America and Europe, people simply open a bottle and take a pill that was made in a factory. Above right: In many other countries, people make medicine at home from plants.

Taking Care of Yourself

Some people do not take care of themselves. They eat too much and do not exercise. They smoke and drink alcohol. When they become ill, they do not go to a doctor right away. When they finally do go to a doctor, they want to be cured quickly. These people may think: "Why should I take care of myself? Medical care is so good that doctors can fix whatever is wrong." Modern medicine cannot cure everything. Many diseases have no cure. Also, medical care can be very costly. Many people do not have that much money.

More and more people want to know how to take good care of themselves so they can stay well. It makes sense to keep illness from happening.

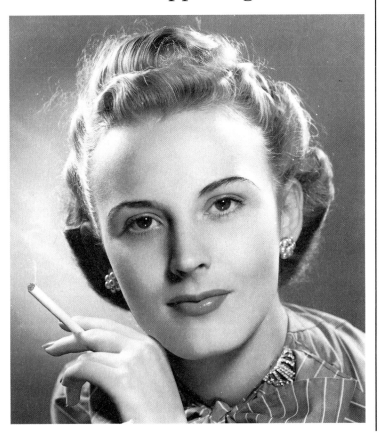

When We Need Medicine

• If you go to bed very late one night, the next day you might not feel very well. This does not mean that you are ill.

• If you have a sore throat and a cough, you might be slightly ill. You may need to rest more than usual. A century ago, people would think you were very healthy!

• If you come down with the flu or the mumps, you are very ill. You will need to stay in bed for several days and be given medical care.

◀ People once thought that smoking was part of being grown-up. But now we know that smoking is bad for a person's health.

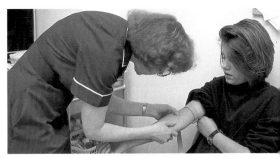

▲ A blood test can warn a person if there is something wrong with his or her health.

Levels of Medical Care

A Chinese doctor checks his patient's pulse to learn more about the illness. Every society has its own way of practicing medicine. ▶

Spending on Health

In the United States, 4.4% of the total budget goes toward health care. Most of this money is spent on diseases, childhood illnesses, veterans, and on health insurance for the poor and elderly.

In the past, people did not know very much about the human body and the things that could go wrong with it. But over time, doctors have learned more about the human body. Today, we have learned so much that a single doctor cannot know everything there is to know about all the different parts of the human

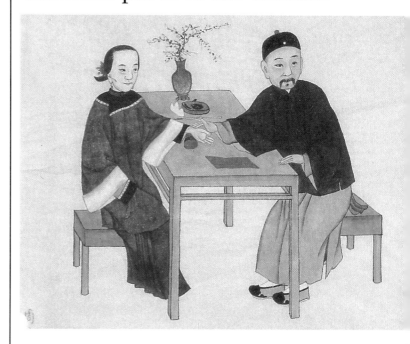

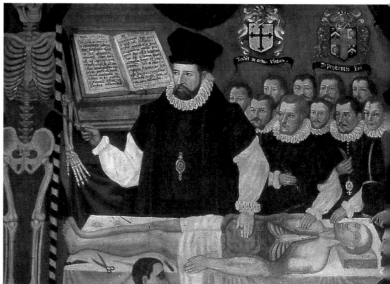

A class in anatomy during the Middle Ages. Even early in history, training doctors took a long time. ▶

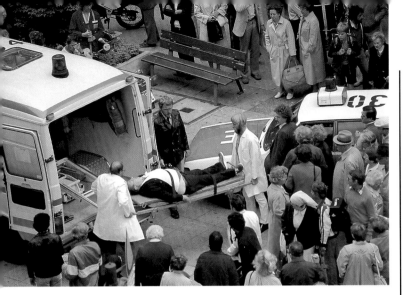

◀ An ambulance crew giving emergency care.

Emergency Care

In a serious accident or disaster, the injured people need medical care right away. A trained ambulance staff gives treatment to the injured. This could be in the form of a fast-acting drug or a splint for a broken leg.

body. So medical help is set up on different levels of care.

Primary Care

The primary care level involves the family doctor. This is the person we usually go to when we are ill. He or she can treat many common illnesses.

Secondary Care

The level of secondary care involves hospitals and specialists. A specialist is a doctor who is an expert in one area of medicine. For example, a pediatrician cares for children. An orthopedic surgeon deals with bones, joints, and muscles. A cardiologist treats heart problems. People go to hospitals for such things as blood tests and x-rays.

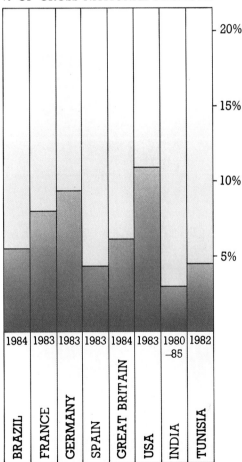

% OF GROSS NATIONAL PRODUCT

BRAZIL	FRANCE	GERMANY	SPAIN	GREAT BRITAIN	USA	INDIA	TUNISIA
1984	1983	1983	1983	1984	1983	1980 –85	1982

▲ How much some countries spend on health care.

2: MEDICINE IN ANCIENT TIMES

Medicine's Beginnings

Medicine began a long, long time ago. It probably started when some people in a tribe or group became more skilled than others at taking care of the sick. Skeletons that are thousands of years old show signs of broken bones. These bones had been set by early healers.

Trepanning

There are also signs of the first medical operations. These signs are neat holes in skulls that are over 10,000 years old. The holes were made during an operation called trepanning. This may have been done to remove evil spirits from the patient.

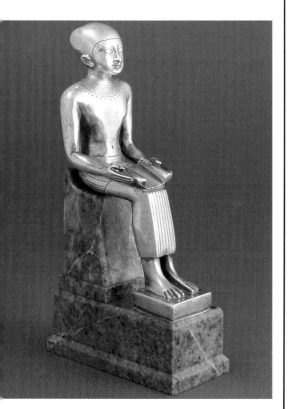

A statue of Imhotep, an early Egyptian doctor.

These ancient stone carvings show some of the surgical instruments used in ancient Egypt. ▶

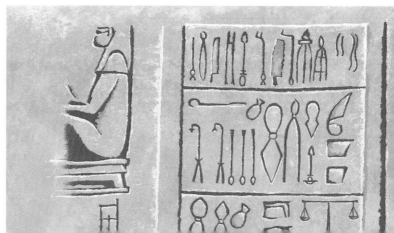

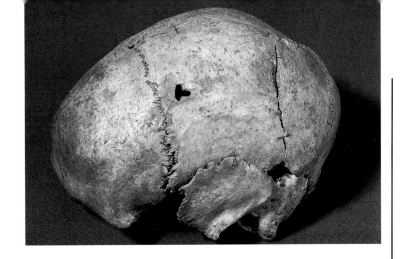

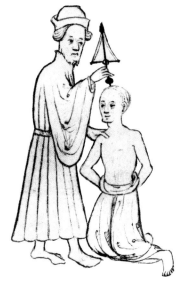

In Ancient Egypt

About 4,600 years ago, a doctor named Imhotep lived in ancient Egypt. People who were sick traveled from very far away so they could be treated by him. After Imhotep died, people made him into a god. People who were ill worshiped statues of him with the hope of being cured. The ancient Egyptians also used medicines. They put moldy bread on their wounds. We now get penicillin from one type of bread mold. The Egyptians also deadened pain with poppy sap, which contains numbing opium.

▲ Above, left: A trepanned hole in a 6,000-year-old skull. Above: Drilling a hole in a skull in the Middle Ages.

Early Medical Writings

Two interesting texts were written on papyrus, a paper made from plants, about 3,500 years ago. The writings tell about medical practices in ancient Egypt.

The Smith papyrus tells how to set broken bones, how to treat eye problems, how to stop bleeding, and how to check a person's pulse. The Ebers papyrus tells how to use about 900 medications. It gives chants and prayers for helping to cure certain illnesses. It also tells about massages, special diets, and hypnosis to help people feel better.

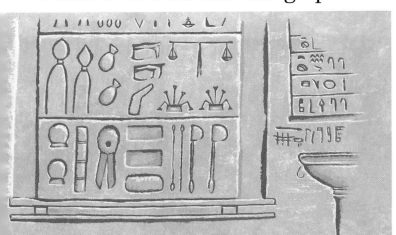

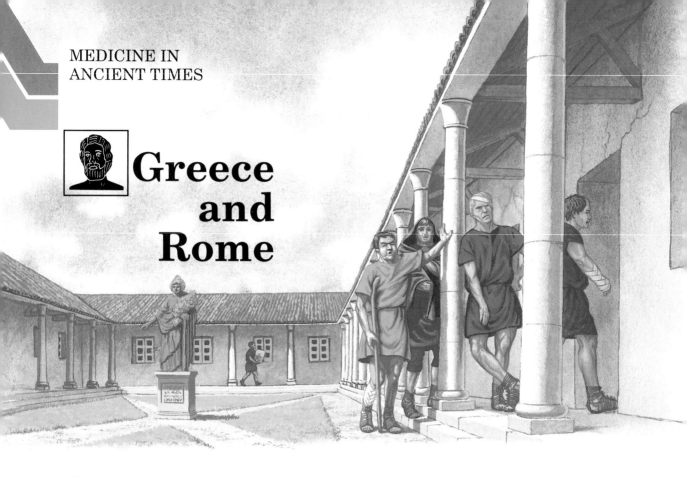

Greece and Rome

▲ One of ancient Rome's *valetudinaria*. These were hospitals where the sick or injured could rest and recover.

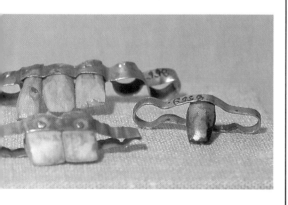

▲ False teeth from ancient Rome. Dental care was only one part of Roman health care.

Ancient Greeks and Romans

In the sixth century BC, Greeks first dissected, or cut open, dead bodies for medical study. Later, they learned that the heart was connected to the blood vessels. Aristotle (born about 384 BC) believed in the scientific method. This means that he made careful observations, did experiments, and carefully noted his findings.

In the first century AD, Celsius wrote an encyclopedia about Roman medicine. The Romans began the first hospitals. They built water systems to make sure that everyone had fresh, clean water. They also got rid of sewage safely. These things helped fight disease.

The Great Galen

Galen (born about AD 130) was a Greek doctor who lived in Rome. He studied the structure and organs of animals, including monkeys. He thought humans were much the same. Galen wrote hundreds of books about the brain, nerves, skeleton, and muscles of the human body.

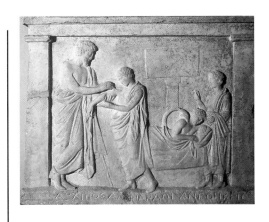

▲ Asklepios treating a patient in the fourth century BC. Ill people prayed for healing in temples built in his honor.

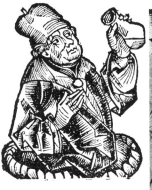

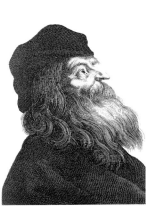

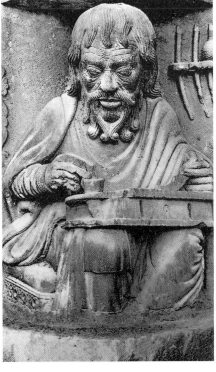

Dreams and Illness

Temples were dedicated to Asklepios, a Greek god of healing. A patient would sleep overnight in one of these temples. Later, the patient would tell a priest about any dreams experienced during the night. The priest would explain the treatment that the dream said the patient needed.

◄ Far left, top: Galen, a doctor of Rome, helped start the study of anatomy. Far left, bottom: Empedocles, of ancient Greece, studied the heart and blood vessels. Left: Aristotle studied comparative anatomy. This is studying and comparing parts of animals.

The Father of Medicine

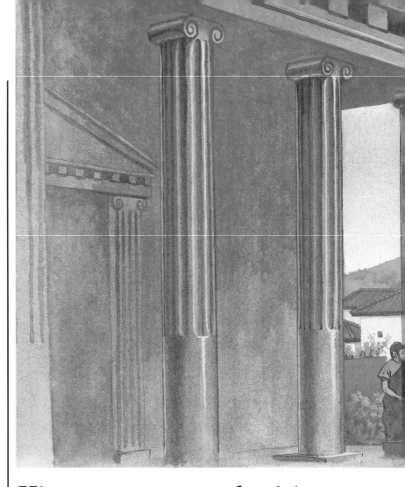

Hippocrates was a physician, a surgeon, and a scientist. He was born about 460 BC on the Greek island of Cos. He was in charge of the hospital and medical school there. His writings and teachings helped found modern medicine. He is often called the Father of Medicine.

In ancient Greece, medicine also included religion and magic. But Hippocrates and his followers did not believe in looking for religious and magic "signs" that caused the illness. Instead, they

Founders of Medicine

Many ancient Greeks and Romans helped to found medicine. But the most famous is Hippocrates.

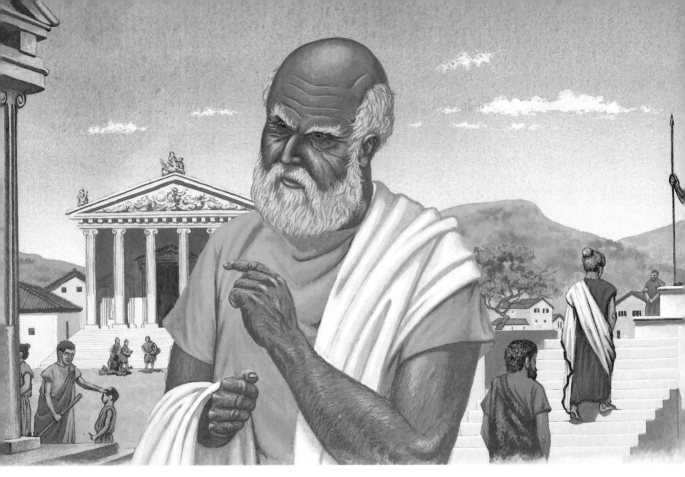

believed that a doctor should examine the patient carefully to identify and treat the illness. They also thought that a doctor should not give any treatment that could harm the patient.

A Moral Code

Hippocrates and his followers developed guidelines about how doctors should think and act. They wrote that a doctor's main job is to help the patient. Also, a doctor should keep secret any personal information he or she finds out about patients.

▲ Hippocrates, as he might have walked through the medical school and hospital on Cos. He taught medicine and encouraged cleanliness.

A Balance
Aristotle believed the body had four "qualities" of hot, cold, wet, and dry, and four "elements" of earth, air, fire, and water. If these got unbalanced, people became ill. Later, this system was replaced by four body "humors" of phlegm, blood, yellow bile, and black bile.

3: MEDIEVAL MEDICINE

Advances under Islam

In Europe, the Middle Ages, or medieval period, lasted from the fifth century to about the fourteenth century. During this time, the medical knowledge and skills of the ancient Egyptians, Romans, and Greeks were forgotten. But in other parts of the world, medical knowledge and practice were expanding.

The Black Death

The Black Death, or bubonic plague, has killed millions of people in the past. Between 1346 and 1350, it killed five million people in Europe alone.

It was called the Black Death partly because bleeding in the skin made dark patches.

This disease is spread by bacteria in two ways: by the bites of fleas that have sucked blood from infected rats, and by droplets coughed up or sneezed out by people. Today, when given early, antibiotics can cure bubonic plague.

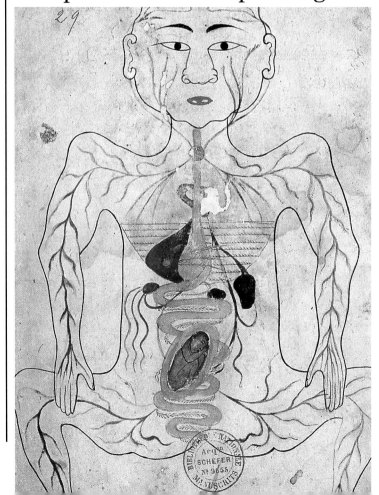

A medical drawing of a pregnant woman made in Persia during the 1100s. ▶

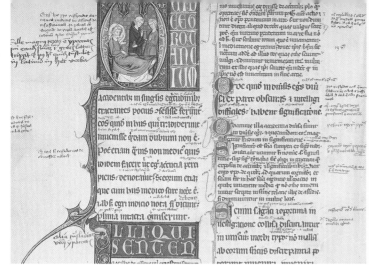

Famous Doctors of Persia

In Persia, now Iran, a doctor known as Rhazes lived until AD 923. Rhazes wrote many medical books and gave one of the first descriptions of the measles. In the early eleventh century, Avicenna, another Persian doctor, wrote *Canon of Medicine*, an encyclopedia. This textbook was used in European medical schools for the next several centuries.

Progress in India

In India, new knowledge about surgical instruments and drugs from medicinal plants was becoming known. A doctor named Susruta believed rightly that mosquitoes could spread the disease malaria and that rats could spread bubonic plague.

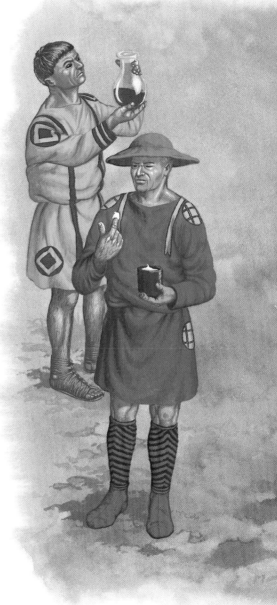

▲ Cosmas and Damian, two saints famous for healing. Many saints were thought to have healing abilities.

Mixing Medicine and Religion

The only hospitals in the Middle Ages were those set up by religious orders. They treated the body and prayed for the soul. ▼

Throughout history, in many parts of the world, medicine has been linked with religion. In the twelfth century, Christianity changed the practice of medicine. Christians during this period thought of illness as being caused by supernatural beings or spirits. Monks used herbs and medicines to treat the sick. But the physical body was considered less important than the state of a person's soul. Prayers and offerings were made to cleanse a sick person's soul. As time went on, the practice of

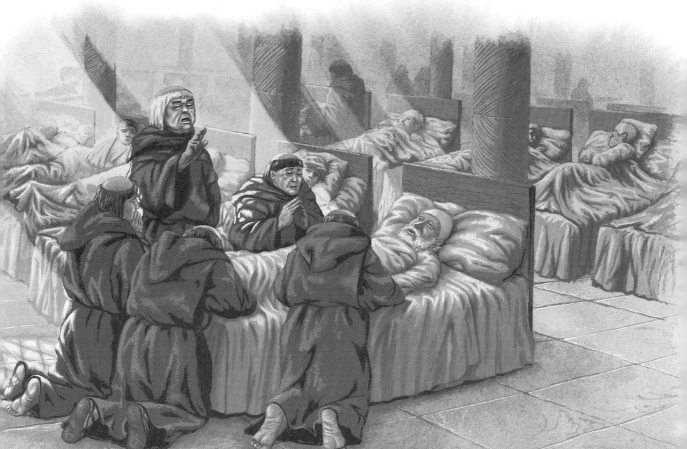

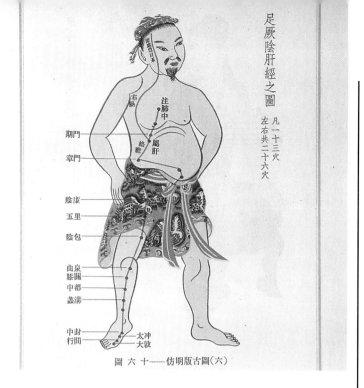

足厥陰肝經之圖

凡一十三穴
左右共二十六穴

右腦
注肺中
屬肝
給膽
期門
章門
陰廉
五里
陰包
曲泉
膝關
中都
蠡溝
中封
行間
太冲
大敦

圖 六 十 ── 仿明版古圖（六）

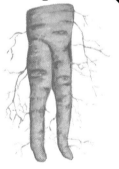

◀ A chart of acupuncture points used in Eastern medicine.

The Doctrine of Signatures

There are many myths, or stories, about the healing powers of plants. Some became part of what is known as the doctrine of signatures. This says that if a plant looks like part of the human body, it can be used to cure that part. For example, lungwort leaves are rounded like lungs, so they were advised for lung disease. The root of meadow saffron looks much like a swollen foot, so doctors used it to treat this condition.

This ginseng root looks like a human's legs. Such likenesses led to the doctrine of signatures. ▼

medicine became mixed with superstitious ideas.

Meanwhile, doctors in the East were learning more and more about medicine. In China, in about 620-30, Chen Ch'uan was probably the first doctor to study diabetes. Beginning in the sixth century, the Chinese wrote a large medical encyclopedia that described over one thousand drugs that helped heal the body.

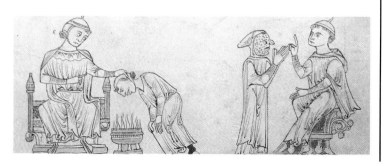

◀ A picture from the 1200s. The patient on the left is getting heat therapy. The one on the right has leprosy.

The Body Structure

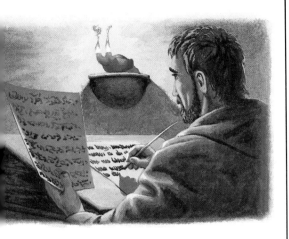

▲ Constantine of Carthage translated Arabic medical works into Latin around 1050-80.

Art and Anatomy

Leonardo da Vinci (1452-1519) was a great artist and a great scientist. He made many detailed drawings of the anatomy of humans and animals. But da Vinci's drawings were not published during his lifetime.

In the third century BC, a Chinese medical book told about human anatomy. In the ninth century, a famous medical school in Salerno, Italy, taught student doctors about anatomy.

The Renaissance

In the early fourteenth century, people became interested in learning new ideas of many kinds. We call this period the Renaissance. Medicine once more began to make progress. Great artists of the time, such as Michelangelo and Leonardo da Vinci, studied the human form.

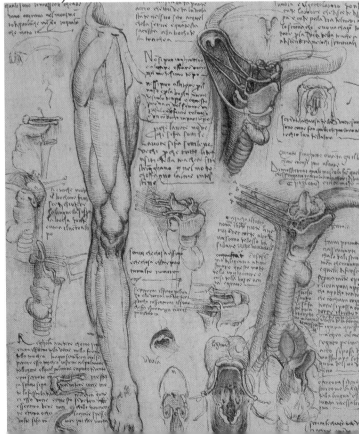

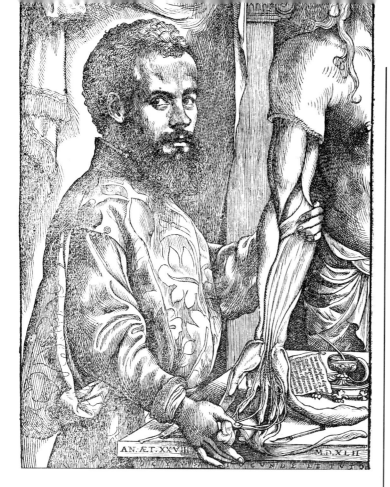

◀ Andreas Vesalius dissects an arm muscle.

The Padua School

The Padua medical school trained many skilled doctors. In the 1500s, Gabriello Fallopio studied the human body in detail. Fallopian tubes in women are named after him.

Santorio Sanctorius, born in 1561, began the study of chemistry. He made instruments to measure body pulse and temperature.

As a result, these artists were able to make correct drawings of the human body.

The Work of Vesalius

Andreas Vesalius was a professor of anatomy and surgery in Italy. He wanted to correct some of Galen's earlier teachings. In 1543, he published a book about human anatomy. Vesalius said that to treat a sick person, a doctor needed to know about the human body's structure and workings when it is healthy.

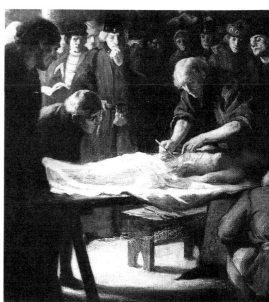

▲ Mondino dei Liucci does a human dissection in 1318.

◀ ◀ Opposite: Leonardo da Vinci's notebook with anatomical drawings.

4: SCIENTIFIC BEGINNINGS

Observation and Experiment

During the seventeenth century, more and more knowledge of medicine became widespread. This was due to the invention of the printing press in the 1400s. The many books printed made it possible for doctors to share their knowledge with each other.

Fernel and Paracelsus

The understanding of anatomy, physiology — how the body works — and disease was increasing all the time. In 1554, Jean François Fernel of France wrote a textbook called *Universa*

Occupational Diseases

Paracelsus thought that a person's job could cause illness, such as a miner developing the disease of miner's lung. One doctor, Bernardino Ramazzini, listed 40 jobs that caused illnesses. He is the founder of what we call occupational medicine.

Right: Paracelsus (1493-1541). ▶

Far right: Jean Fernel (1506-88). ▶

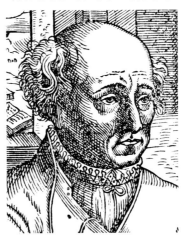
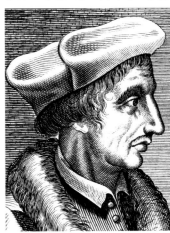

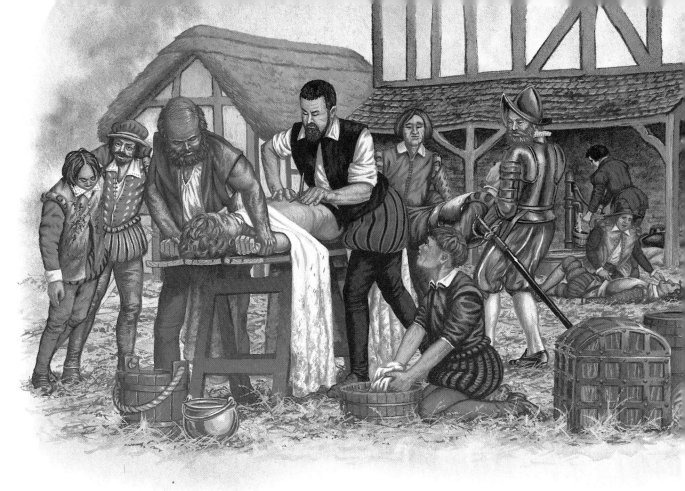

Medicina. It had a lot of new information about the anatomy of humans, their physiology, treatments, and pathology — the study of diseased organs.

About the same time, a doctor called Paracelsus was treating people in Europe. He helped his patients with new chemical drugs that were made of lead, mercury, sulfur, antimony, iron, and copper. He also felt that it was helpful for patients to talk about their illnesses.

Ambroise Paré, army surgeon and doctor to four French kings in the 1600s.

Infectious Diseases

Through the centuries, some doctors thought that germs might cause some diseases. Girolamo Fracastoro, an Italian doctor, said in 1546 that disease could spread in three ways: (1) by touching the ill person's body, (2) by touching something the ill person had already touched, and (3) by being in the same place as the ill person.

Medical Advances

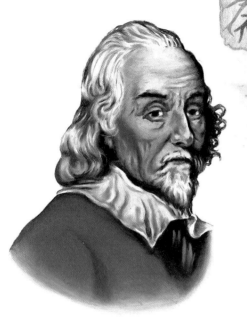

▲ William Harvey saw how the heart's valves controlled the flow of blood, like valves used in machines at the time.

Opposite, top: Thomas Sydenham studied the diagnosis of disease. ▶ ▶

Opposite, bottom: Pierre Fauchard made dentistry a specialty. ▶ ▶

Medical doctors once thought that the blood was made in the liver and that the heart warmed it. The blood was thought to seep from veins to arteries through little holes in the heart's wall. The heartbeat and pulse were said to be caused by the blood going back and forth in the blood vessels. Some time later, however, Italian doctors showed that blood could not seep through the heart's wall. But they could not explain what happened to it instead.

William Harvey

In 1628, William Harvey, an English doctor, discovered that blood flows continuously around the body in just one direction. The heart pumps the blood, and valves keep the blood flowing only one way. But Harvey could not explain how the blood went from the small arteries into the small veins.

Thomas Sydenham

Thomas Sydenham was known as the English Hippocrates. He wrote a book in 1666, called *The Method of Treating Fevers*. Sydenham believed that doctors should help guide the body's own healing powers. His notes on the case histories of his patients are still admired today.

Pierre Fauchard

The Chinese had been filling and capping teeth for centuries. In Europe, French doctor Pierre Fauchard was the first to think of dentistry as a specialty of medicine. In 1728, he wrote *The Surgeon Dentist*.

Did You Know?

Today, taking a person's pulse is common. John Floyer, an English doctor, discovered that the pulse rate could be used to find out about a person's health. He told of this discovery in 1707.

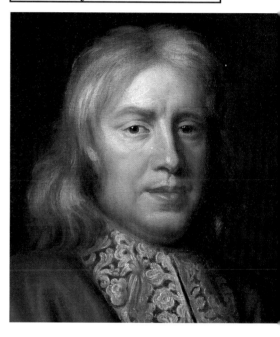

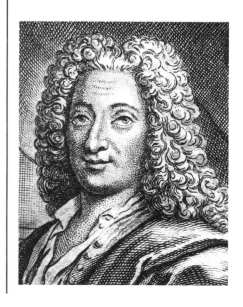

Medicine Branches Out

Edward Jenner

Edward Jenner was a doctor who had the idea of vaccination — giving someone weak germs so the body prepares to fight against getting a worse disease. Jenner knew that people who had the disease cowpox would not later catch a more serious disease called smallpox. In 1796, he proved this to be true.

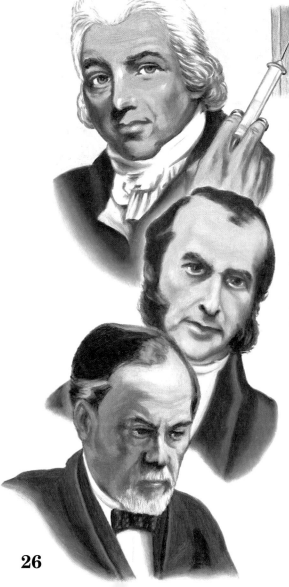

Thomas Hodgkin

Thomas Hodgkin specialized in pathology, the study of diseased organs. His work in the early 1800s helped make pathology an important part of medicine.

Louis Pasteur

In the mid-1800s, Louis Pasteur, a French chemist, showed that changes such as the souring of milk came from the action of tiny living things. He proved that these germs floated in the air or traveled on objects. He found ways to prevent infections.

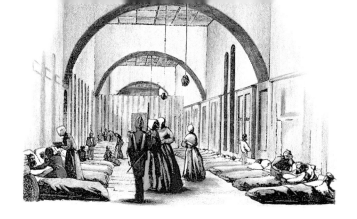

Florence Nightingale

Florence Nightingale was the founder of nursing. She helped care for British soldiers who were wounded in war. Florence Nightingale developed new methods in nursing. She began the first nursing school in 1860.

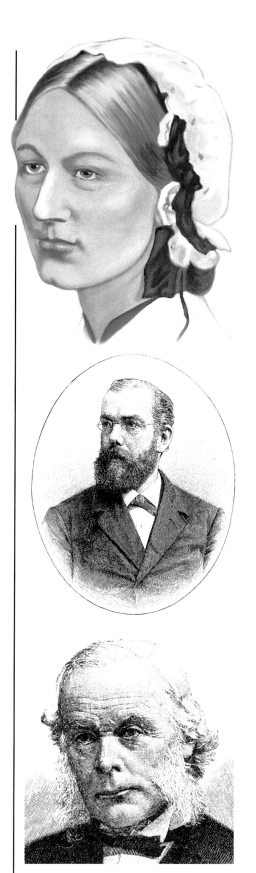

Joseph Lister

Joseph Lister made surgery much safer by fighting infection in patients. In the mid-1800s, he was the first to use chemicals called antiseptics to kill the organisms that cause infection.

Robert Koch

Robert Koch started the science of bacteriology. He showed that bacteria are the cause of many infectious diseases. He grew and studied them. In 1882, he discovered the bacteria that causes the disease tuberculosis.

Microscopes and Medicine

Marcello Malpighi, an Italian, was the first doctor to use a microscope. In 1661, while looking at a frog's lung under a microscope, he saw the capillaries that connect arteries and veins. This completed the blood circuit described by Harvey. Malpighi studied eggs, helping found the science of embryology.

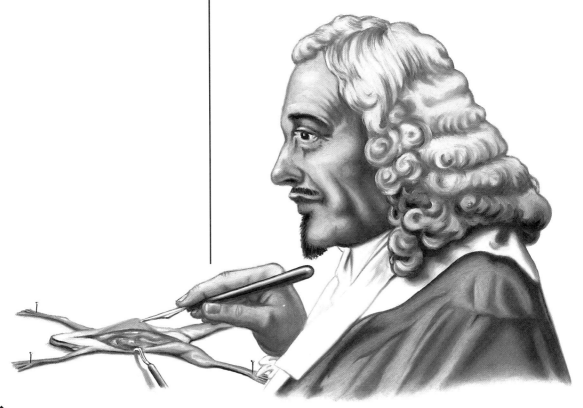

▲ Marcello Malpighi studies the microscopic structure of frog tissues. Tubes that help the bodies of some animals get rid of wastes are named malpighian tubules after him.

Anton van Leeuwenhoek, a Dutch clothing dealer, had no scientific training. Yet he made his own microscopes with lenses he ground himself. In the 1600s,

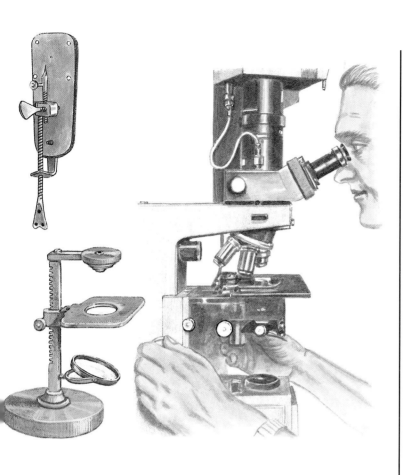

◀ Far left, top: Anton van Leeuwenhoek's first microscope, a hand-held model. Far left, bottom: A later table-top model by Leeuwenhoek. Left: A modern electron microscope that can see tiny details inside cells.

he described and drew pictures of red blood cells, muscle fibers, and harmless bacteria that he saw. Gradually, doctors began to use the microscope to help diagnose and treat disease. In the late 1800s, microscopes were greatly improved.

The Cell Theory

By the middle of the nineteenth century, scientists discovered that all living things were made up of tiny living units. They called these living units cells.

Cellular Pathology

A Prussian doctor, Rudolf Virchow, was certain that body tissues were made up of cells and their products. He said that every cell in the body had been made from a cell that existed before. Virchow also believed that people get diseases when cells work the wrong way, or are being destroyed. These changes can be seen with a microscope. His ideas led to the founding of the branch of medicine called cellular pathology.

5: A TIME OF PROGRESS

Insects and Disease

Frederick Banting and Charles Best, of Canada, with the first dog they injected with insulin in 1921. Insulin became the treatment for diabetes. ▼

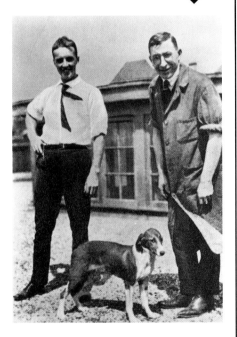

In 1900, American army doctor Walter Reed led a team that showed that the disease yellow fever was spread by the bite of a mosquito. Clearing away areas where mosquitoes bred checked the spread of yellow fever. Also in 1900, a Scottish military officer, William Leishman, found that the tropical disease kala-azar (now known as leishmaniasis) was spread by sand flies.

This psychiatric patient is being treated with art therapy. This is when painting and drawing may help heal a patient who is having mental or emotional problems. ▶

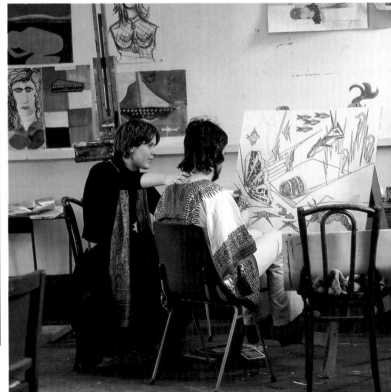

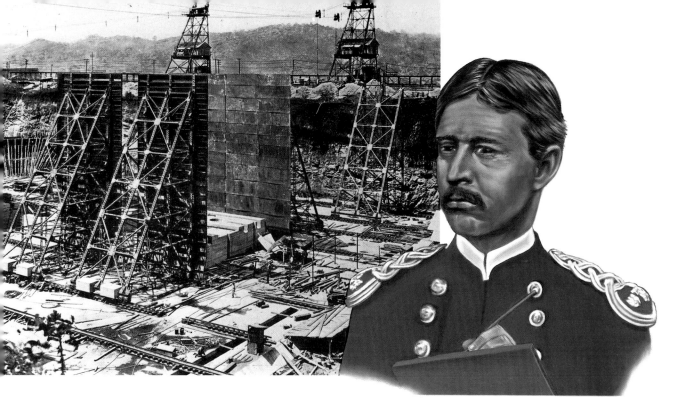

Blood Groups

Karl Landsteiner, an Austrian doctor, showed in 1900 that not all human blood was the same. He found groups A, B, O, and AB. In 1940, Landsteiner found the Rhesus, or Rh, blood types.

Mental Illness

Sigmund Freud, an Austrian doctor, developed the main ideas of psychiatry. Psychiatry deals with illnesses of the mind.

Medical Teams

The time of a lone doctor making discoveries began to end. From then on, doctors started to work together in research teams.

▲ Walter Reed learned how to control yellow fever. This made life safer for the men building the Panama Canal, seen in the background.

Modern Drugs

In 1908, Paul Ehrlich, a German bacteriologist, won the Nobel Prize for medicine. He studied the way the body fights disease. He vaccinated children against the disease diphtheria. In 1910, Ehrlich made a drug in his laboratory for treating the disease syphilis. This was the start of modern drug therapy, with medicines made from chemicals, instead of coming from plants or animals.

The First Antibiotic

Alexander Fleming checks the growth of bacteria in a culture plate. ▶

Tropical swamps like this one are home to the *Anopheles* mosquito. This mosquito spreads malaria with its bite. ▼

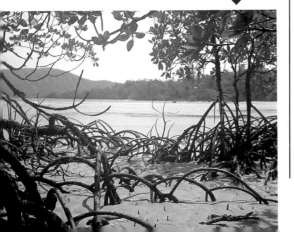

In 1928, an accident caused one of the greatest advances in medicine. Alexander Fleming, a British scientist, was studying bacteria in his laboratory. He was growing the bacteria in the usual way, in round dishes called culture plates. Some mold got into one of the plates. As the mold grew, it killed the bacteria. Fleming found that a substance made by the mold could kill several types of bacteria that caused infections. Fleming called this substance made by the mold penicillin.

Production and Testing

The next job was to make pure penicillin in large amounts. The first tests of penicillin during World War II were successful. This was the beginning of the era of antibiotic drugs.

Antibiotics Today

Today, there are dozens of antibiotic drugs, with new ones appearing all the time. Some antibiotics kill only a few types of bacteria. Others attack many types of bacteria.

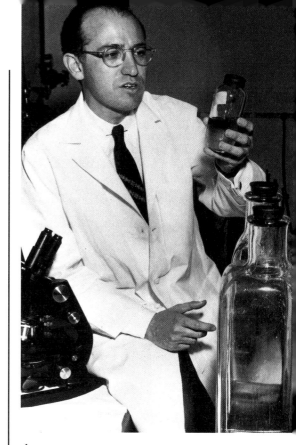

Jonas Salk examines microbe-culture bottles. He developed the first vaccine against polio, a crippling disease.

Did You Know?

Malaria is one of the world's major diseases. Starting in 1630, the drug quinine was used to treat it. Quinine comes from the cinchona tree. From about 1934, human-made drugs have been used to fight malaria.

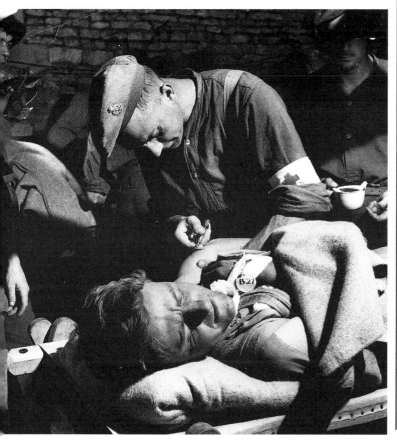

◀ Injured troops getting antibiotic injections during World War II. This saved many lives.

33

Advances in Surgery

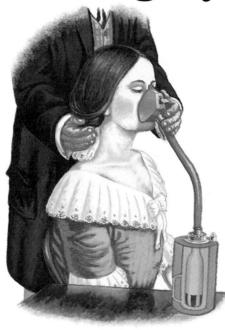

▲ This type of chloroform inhaler was used to put patients to sleep in the 1850s by John Snow, an anesthetist in Britain.

William Morton, a dentist, using ether as an anesthetic at Massachusetts General Hospital in 1846. ▶

Many improvements in surgery were made during the first fifty years of the 1900s. This was partly because of anesthesia. Anesthesia makes a patient feel no pain when having surgery.

Anesthetics

Early doctors gave their patients drugs to dull the patient's senses during surgery. But there were no drugs then that would put a patient completely to sleep. This meant that surgery had to be done quickly. In 1845, a dentist, Horace Wells, used the gas nitrous oxide to make pulling

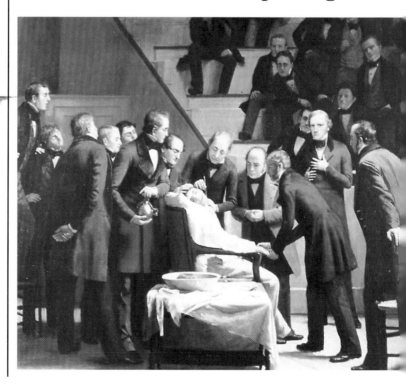

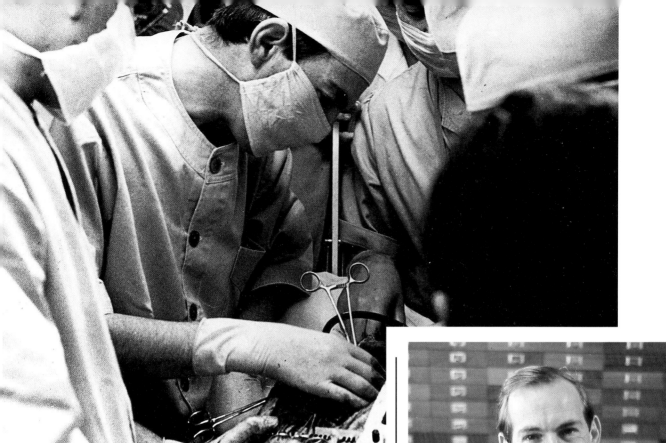

teeth painless. In 1846, another dentist, William Morton, used ether fumes to put a patient to sleep. Then Dr. John C. Warren operated painlessly on the neck of the patient. By 1847, doctors were using chloroform as an anesthetic. Since that time, anesthesia has become an important part of medicine. Anesthesia allows doctors to take more time during surgery and use better methods, because the patient cannot feel any pain.

▲ Top: Dr. Christiaan Barnard operating on an anesthetized patient.
Above: Dr. Barnard did the first heart transplant.

X-rays and Radiology

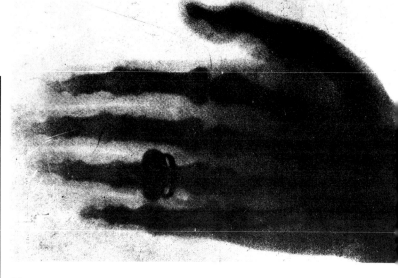

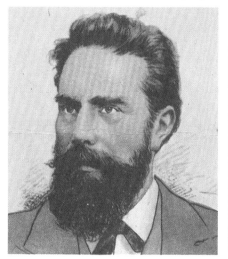

Above: Wilhelm Röntgen. Above, top: Wilhelm Röntgen's x-ray of his wife's hand shows her bones and ring.

An x-ray clinic of the late 1800s. The dangers of x-rays were unknown then, so no one wore protective clothing. ▶

In 1895, Wilhelm Röntgen was experimenting with a device called the vacuum tube. He found that it gave off invisible rays that could pass through flesh but not bone. He called these rays x-rays.

Doctors soon began using x-ray pictures to look at organs inside

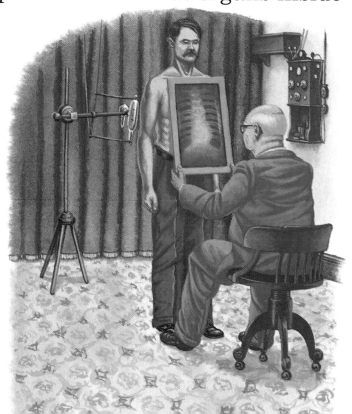

Did You Know?

The first patient helped by x-rays was Eddie McCarthy, an American. In 1896, his broken arm was x-rayed and set.

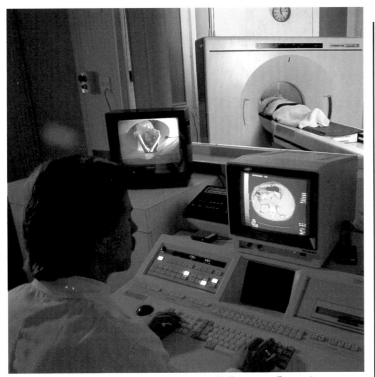

◀ A CAT scan taking place. A complete cross section of the patient's body shows up on the monitor screen.

Dangerous X-rays

During the early days of x-rays, some workers suffered from skin ulcers, anemia, and cancer. It was later proved that high doses of x-rays harmed living tissues and brought on disease. Today, doctors can use carefully controlled doses of radiation to kill off diseased tissues such as cancer. This is known as radiotherapy.

the body and to find breaks in bones. In the early 1900s, a method was developed to make an x-ray of the digestive system. In 1922, a similar method was developed to make an x-ray of a person's lungs.

The use of x-rays grew into a branch of medicine called radiology. The CAT scan connects x-rays with computers to make a complete picture of a patient's insides. Today, we have other ways of seeing inside the body. These modern methods include the use of heat, sound waves, and electromagnetism.

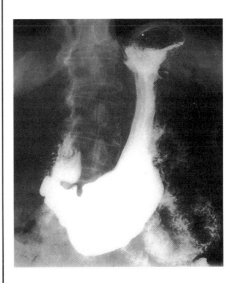

▲ An x-ray of a stomach. The patient swallows a substance that shows the stomach as white.

6: | MEDICINE TODAY

Checkups and Tests

This girl is having her six-month dental checkup. The dentist looks for signs of tooth decay and gum disease, then cleans the teeth. ▶

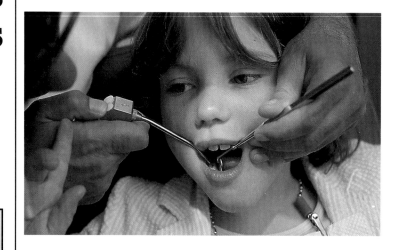

The Quality of Life

Treatment that helps people live longer does not always stop their suffering. For example, a baby may be born deformed. Many operations may be needed to help the baby survive. But the baby's life may not be good. An elderly person may have a serious disease that could be cured with treatment. But the treatment has terrible side effects, and again, the quality of life would not be good. The patients, their relatives, and their doctors must decide if treatment will help the patients lead useful lives without too much pain.

Screening Tests

Doctors have many ways to search for diseases in a person who seems to be well. This is called screening or having a checkup. But doctors cannot screen for every illness. So they look for certain serious diseases, such as some cancers and heart problems that have early warning signs. Screening is usually done on people who are at the most risk. These may be old people, or the very young, or persons with a family history of disease, or men only, or women.

Diagnostic Tests

When an ill person visits the doctor, he or she will take the patient's medical history. The doctor asks about symptoms and about the patient's past health. Next, the doctor and medical staff may carry out blood, urine, or other diagnostic tests to find out the cause of the illness.

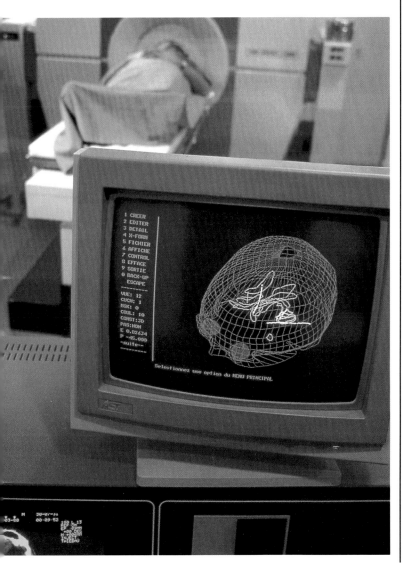

◄ A CAT scanner reveals a brain tumor. The computer screen shows the tumor in green lines.

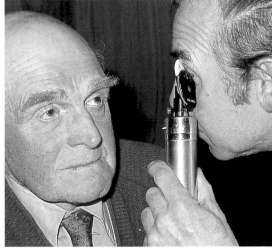

▲ A doctor looks at the blood vessels and nerves inside a patient's eye. Problems like high blood pressure can show up.

Electronic Eyes

Below: Thermography measures the heat of body parts. This can show unhealthy growths. Below right: Nuclear magnetic resonance (NMR) uses magnets to make an image. Bottom right: The NMR shows tissues clearly. ▼

ECGs and EEGs

As the heart pumps and the brain thinks, they send out tiny bursts of electricity. The ECG, or electrocardiograph, shows the heart's beating as wavy lines on a chart. These can tell the doctor if the heart is diseased. The EEG, or electroencephalograph, shows the brain's waves, or signals. These brain waves can tell a doctor if the brain has been injured or is not working normally. Today, doctors use many machines to help them look inside the body. They can

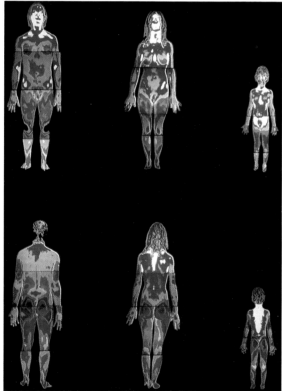

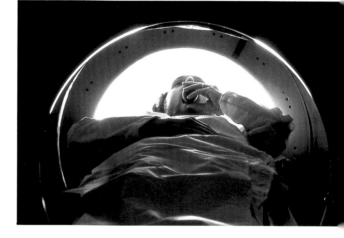

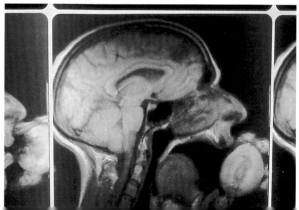

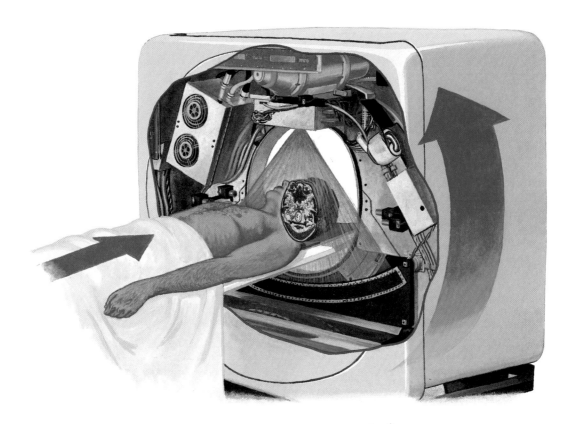

see the structure and workings of organs such as the kidneys and liver without cutting the body open. This helps doctors find and treat diseases before they become too serious. Images from inside the body are getting better all the time.

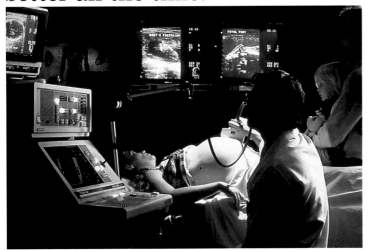

◀ This pregnant woman is having an ultrasound scan. High-pitched sound waves are sent through her body. The sound waves are then turned into an image by a computer. Ultrasound helps to check if a developing baby is healthy.

41

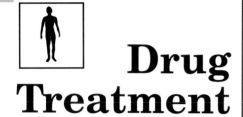

Drug Treatment

There are thousands of drugs in use in the medical field today. Some are from natural sources, such as plants. But most drugs are now made in laboratories. Dozens of new drugs are made available to people each year.

Prescribing Drugs

Prescribing, or ordering, the correct drug for a patient is not easy. It must be the right drug to treat that disease. The dose, or amount, must be right for the person. The patient must not have any condition that would cause problems. For example, some drugs should not be given to a patient who has kidney

Developing a new drug takes years and costs a great deal of money. Only a few of the many drugs tested pass all the tests and go on sale. ▼

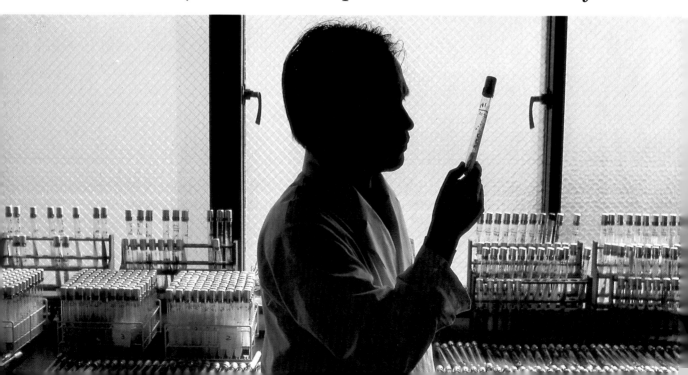

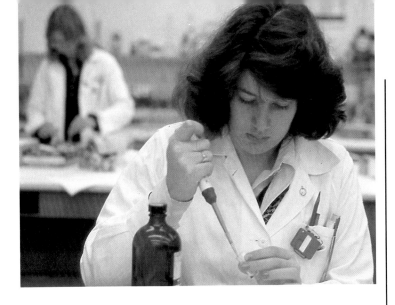

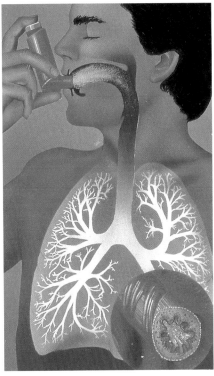

◀ Tests done on samples of blood, urine, and other body fluids show how the body breaks down the drug. This can tell how the drug is working.

disease. Some people might be allergic to a drug. Taking more than one drug at a time may also cause problems. A new drug has to pass many tests before people can start to use it. Sometimes a problem shows up years after the drug has been in use. Then doctors no longer give that drug to their patients.

▲ A drug for controlling asthma is sprayed into the lungs as a fine mist. This is an example of a drug going to the right place quickly in order to help the patient.

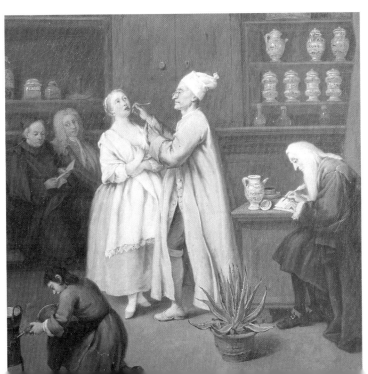

◀ The old-time apothecary, or drug store, sold minerals and parts of plants and animals to help cure illness. But doctors did not know how these drugs worked in the body.

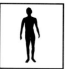

New Body Parts

Most surgeons specialize in one area of the body. The cardiac surgeon operates on the heart. The neurosurgeon operates on the brain and nerves. Surgeons are helped by other surgeons, the anesthetist, nurses, and people using special equipment, like the heart-lung machine.

Transplants

A transplant is a part of one person's body that is put into the body of another person. Body parts that can be transplanted include the heart, lungs, liver, kidneys, pancreas, bone marrow,

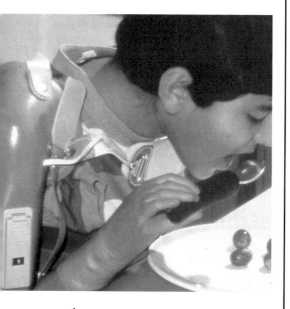

▲ This boy is learning to use an artificial arm. It works by sensing the electrical signals from the boy's muscles. These signals move the arm in the way the boy wants.

One type of heart valve (inset) and an x-ray of this valve inside a living heart. ▶

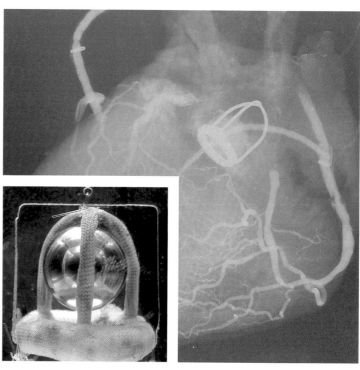

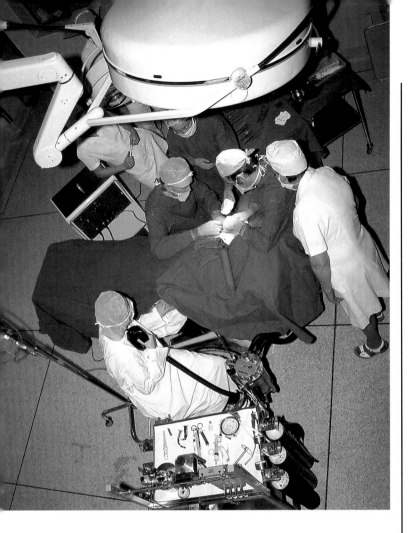

◀ A surgical team. Surgeons and nurses surround the patient. The anesthetist is near the bottom.

Transplants and Implants

1. Metal plate	15. Elbow joint
2. Plastic eye	16. Wrist joint
3. Artificial ear	17. Knuckles
4. Bridge anchor	18. Liver
5. Jaw	19. Kidney
6. Teeth	20. Pancreas
7. Voice box	21. Insulin pump
8. Lung	
9. Arm	22. Hip joint
10. Pacemaker	23. Metal thighbone
11. Valve	
12. Heart	24. Knee
13. Breast implant	25. Metal shin
14. Shoulder joint	26. Leg

and many others. Sometimes the patient's body will reject, or fight against, the transplant. Certain drugs can help keep this from happening.

Implants

Artificial, or human-made, body parts are called implants. False teeth, wooden legs, and glass eyes have been used for a long time. Today, many new types of implants, such as pacemakers and artificial hips, are in use.

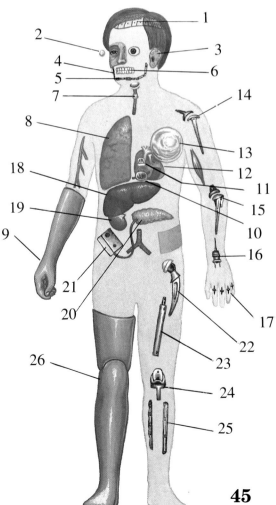

45

Treating the Mind

The ancient Chinese, Greeks, and Indians knew that some illnesses seemed to be caused by something in the ill person's mind. Early ideas of mental illness were often linked to magic, superstition, and evil spirits. For centuries during the Middle Ages, people with mental illness were locked away and forgotten. There was no treatment and little hope of them getting well.

Worries about jobs and getting along with people can strain mental health in a person already troubled with, for example, a poor self-image or goals that are too high to reach. If left untreated, these can lead to mental problems. ▶

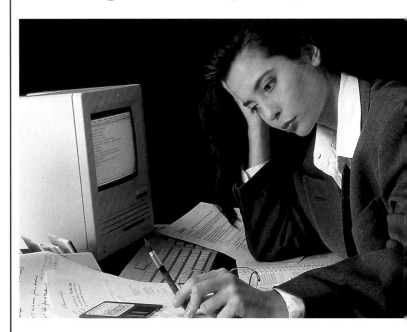

Psychiatry

In the late nineteenth and early twentieth centuries, several doctors became interested in mental illness. One of the first was Sigmund Freud, a doctor from Vienna, Austria. Freud studied how the mind works and why people behave as they do. He found a method called psychoanalysis to treat his mentally ill patients. Later doctors found other kinds of treatment, including the use of drugs. Psychiatry has become a major branch of medicine. New studies tell us that some kinds of mental illness can come from physical problems in the human brain.

What Is Mental Illness?

Most people can handle life's ups and downs. But sometimes, if a person's mind already carries heavy problems, handling the stresses of daily life can then become difficult.

In a mental illness, a person's mind and thinking are no longer normal. He or she cannot handle daily life very well. The person may have odd moods and act strangely.

If the patient knows that there is a problem, and the illness is not too serious, it is called a neurosis. But a person with a psychosis loses touch with the world and does not know that there is something wrong.

◀ Sigmund Freud founded psychoanalysis. He said that by facing our buried thoughts, we could overcome our mental and emotional problems.

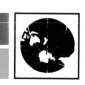

7: MEDICINE IN OTHER PLACES

China

Chinese medicine is probably the oldest in the world. In China, people believe that health is based on the harmony, or agreement, of opposite forces. These forces are called *yin* and *yang*. Illness happens when the two forces are out of balance. One way to restore this energy balance is by using acupuncture. Needles are placed in certain points of the body to slow or speed the energy. Other treatments include herbs, massage, and special exercises.

Barefoot Doctors

In China, there are not enough doctors to go around. "Barefoot

▲ The symbol for yin and yang. Traditional Chinese medicine balances these opposite forces to bring about good health.

Traditional medicines for sale in a street market in China. Many sellers know how to make and use these ancient remedies. ▶

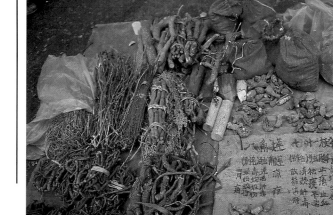

doctors" are health workers with some training. They teach the people hygiene and treat their common illnesses.

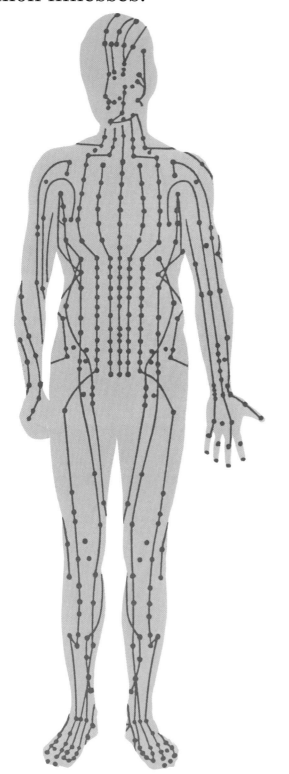

Medical Facts: China

• People lived about 30 years in 1949, but 70 years today. Of every 1,000 babies born, 35 die.

• There is one doctor for every 2,000 people and one hospital bed for every 500 people.

North America:

• People live about 76 years. Of every 1,000 babies born, eight die.

• There is one doctor for every 452 people and one hospital bed for every 156 people.

◀ Acupuncture channels carry the body's energy. Needles put into the body at certain points speed up or slow down the energy.

▼ Putting acupuncture needles in a patient's scalp.

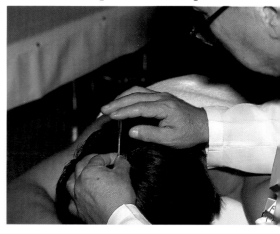

India and the Middle East

Health workers in India ▶
tell people about birth
control. Too many people
means not enough food,
water, sewer lines, and
health services to go
around.

Medical Facts: India

• People live for 58 years.

• Of every 1,000 babies
born, 110 die.

• India sees birth control
as the way to control its
population growth.

• There is one doctor for
every 3,600 people and
one hospital bed for every
1,600 people.

Shantytowns in India have
open sewers and dirty
water. Flies spread germs
that cause disease. ▶

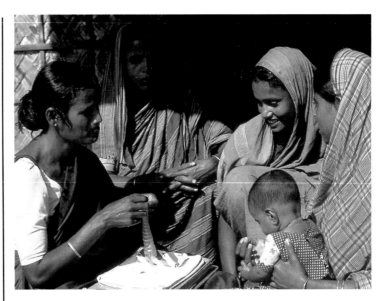

India and Pakistan

In both India and Pakistan, the
traditional medicine is several
thousand years old. It is based
on herbs and other medicinal
substances. Most doctors in
India and Pakistan are trained
in both traditional and Western-
style medicine.

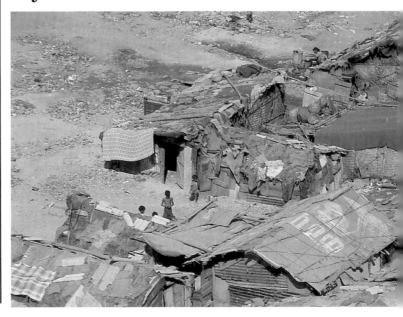

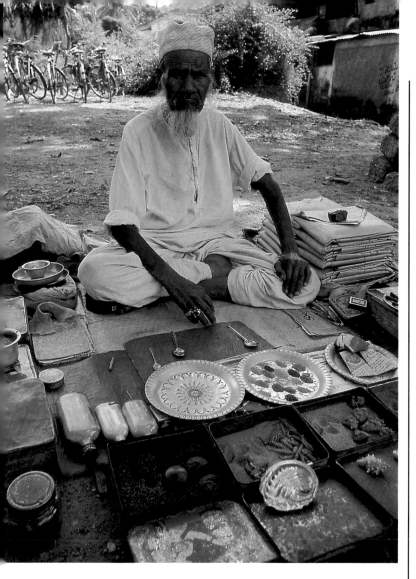

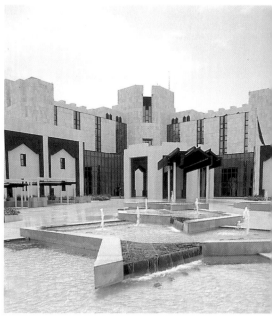

◀ A man sells traditional medicines on a street in India. He can give advice about which herbs to use for different illnesses.

▲ The King Khalid Eye Hospital in Saudi Arabia. Money from selling oil built this hospital.

The Middle East

Some of the countries of the Middle East have become rich from selling oil. These countries can pay for modern sanitation and Western-style medicine. But other Middle East countries are very poor. They do not have safe sewage disposal or clean water. In these countries, the people suffer from many illnesses that can be prevented.

The herb rauwolfia has been used for over 2,000 years in India. It can calm a person's nerves and lower his or her blood pressure. ▼

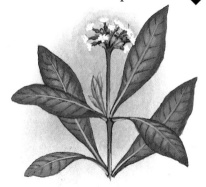

Africa

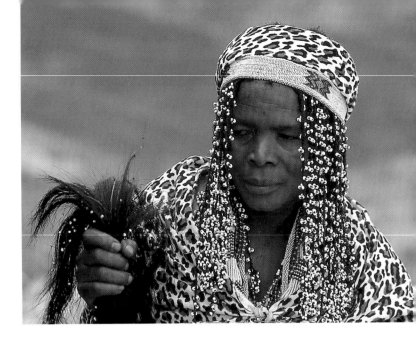

An African spirit healer. ▶
She holds a special object
that helps her use her
spiritual powers.

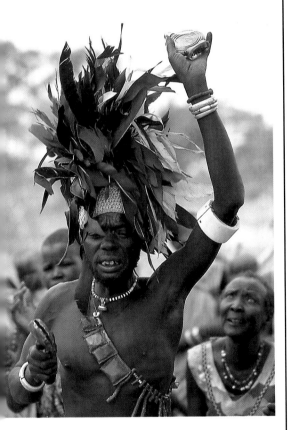

▲ A traditional African
healer, holding a bottle
of medicine during a
healing ceremony.

Healing by the Spirits

Traditional medicine in Africa is
practiced by a healer, usually a
man. He can make medicines
from plants and animal parts.
He can gain power from the
spirits, so he is able to cure the
sick. In some countries, these
healers have become part of the
government medical system.

Problems and Goals

The causes of illness in Africa
are mainly lack of food, poverty,
and unclean conditions. Health
care workers in Africa try to control diseases such as malaria, to
grow enough food for everyone to
eat well, to cure diseases with
drugs, and to vaccinate children
against childhood diseases.

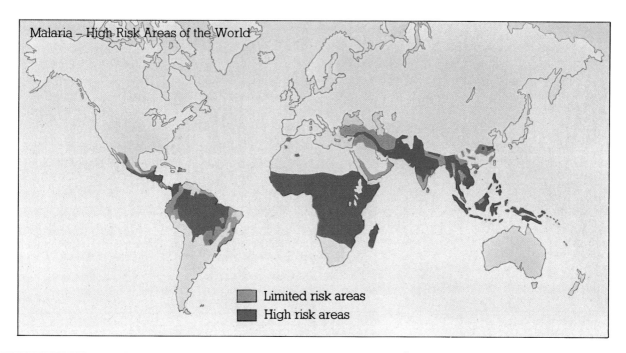

Malaria – High Risk Areas of the World

Limited risk areas
High risk areas

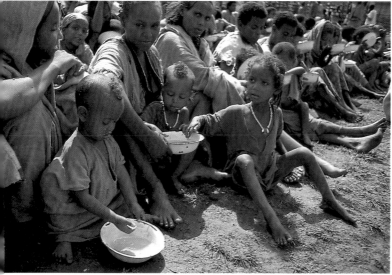

▲ Malaria is one of the world's most serious health problems.

◀ These children from Ethiopia are starving. The food crops dried up because there was no rain. When people starve, they become ill very easily.

Where and Who You Are

In Africa, sick people are often far away from medical care. Some may be refused care because of their race or the group they belong to. Some sick people may be too poor to pay for any kind of medical treatment.

Medical Facts: Kenya

• Women live an average 61 years; men, 57.

• For every 1,000 babies born, 50 die.

• There is one doctor for every 10,000 people and one hospital bed for every 1,000 people.

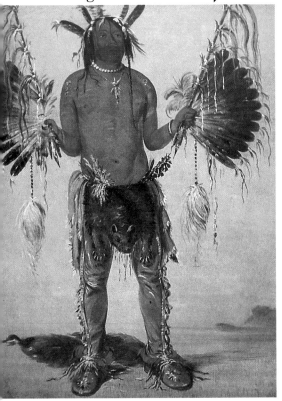

The Americas

This man from Ecuador grows herbs for medicine high in the Andes. ▶

▲ The Mandan medicine man, a Native American healer painted in 1832 by the artist George Catlin.

Native American Traditions

Many American Indians believe that illness is due to forces from the spirit world. These forces are tied closely to nature.

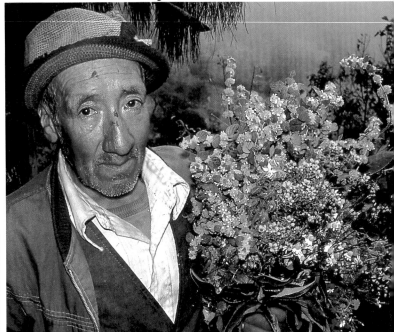

When a North American Indian became ill, the first person to see was the group's herbalist. This herbalist gave certain herbs to the ill person to take to cure the sickness. Sometimes, the spirit healer of the tribe would also be called upon. This healer would smoke, sniff, or chew certain plants that contain drugs. The healer went into a trance and talked with spirits in order to heal the person's illness.

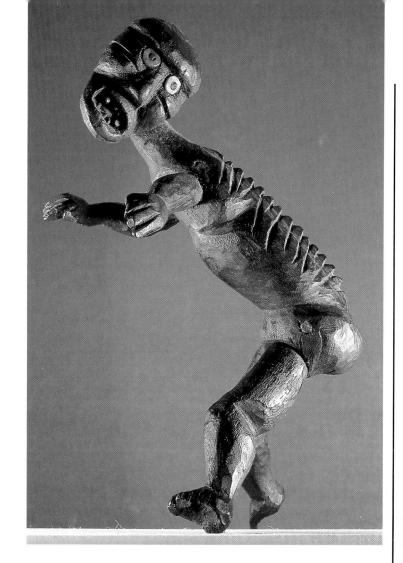

◀ Some Inuit from North America make small statues as offerings to the spirits for a long and healthy life.

Medical Facts: Brazil

• Women live an average of 67 years; men, 62.

• Of every 1,000 babies born, fewer than 70 die.

• There is one doctor for every 2,300 people and one hospital bed for 280.

Medical Facts: Bolivia

• People live 50 years.

• Of every 1,000 babies born, over 120 die.

South American Traditions

The Indians of South America also use herbs for healing. One famous group of healers is the Kallawaya from Bolivia. They travel with bags of dried herbs, diagnosing and treating illness and carrying out healing rituals. Many of our modern medicines first came from traditional herbs used by the Indians of North and South America. Later, we found ways to make them.

Did You Know?

When Cortez invaded Mexico in 1520, his army brought diseases like smallpox and measles. These diseases were new to the Indians, and their bodies could not fight them. Over 50 million Indians died of disease in the century after Europeans came to the Americas.

8: MEDICINE IN THE FUTURE

The Coming Challenges

Medicine continues to face many challenges. Some diseases, like malaria, have been around since history began. Others, such as AIDS, are new.

Environmental Illness

Each year, about six million people in the world develop cancer. In cancer, body cells multiply and form growths. For a long time, the causes of cancer were a mystery. But now cancer is being linked with the environment. Certain foods and too much sunshine can also cause cancer. And some chemicals can start cancer in the body.

Clean air, good food, and pure water are needed for health. We may someday find that today's air pollution has caused diseases that take years to show up in humans. ▶

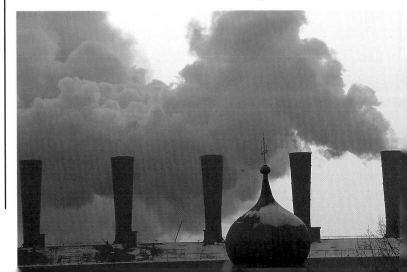

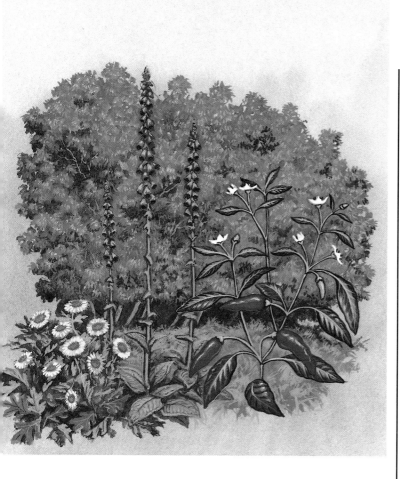

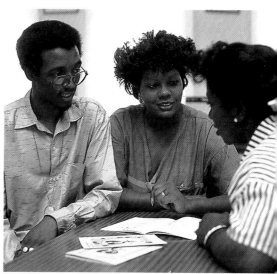

The foxglove flower in the center contains medicines that help the heart beat more smoothly and regularly. This was discovered by William Withering, an English doctor of the 1700s.

Certain diseases run in families and in some ethnic groups. Medical specialists can decide if future children are likely to get one of these diseases.

A New Disease

In the early 1980s, doctors found a new disease — acquired immune deficiency syndrome (AIDS). It is caused by human immunodeficiency virus (HIV). Many people have died from AIDS. Millions of people carry the HIV virus. Scientists are still learning about this virus. They are trying to find better treatments, a vaccine, and even a cure for AIDS. Research on AIDS has helped scientists learn more about the human body.

Better Treatment

In the 1950s, only one child in 25 was cured of the blood cancer acute lymphatic leukemia. By the late 1970s, one child in two was cured. This happened because the disease could be found earlier and better treatments could be given for it.

Healing the World

These children in Romania have AIDS. They get little medical care and do not have modern hospitals or the latest medicines to help them live better or longer. ▶

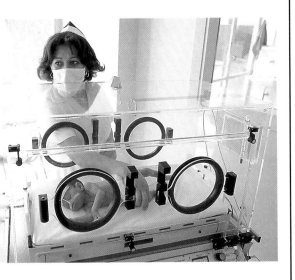

▲ A newborn British baby in an incubator. This baby is getting the best care in a modern hospital that has the latest equipment.

Prevention Is Best

All people need good food, clean water, safe waste disposal, and good living conditions. Wars, religion, and politics can make it harder to have these. In richer countries, people are learning to

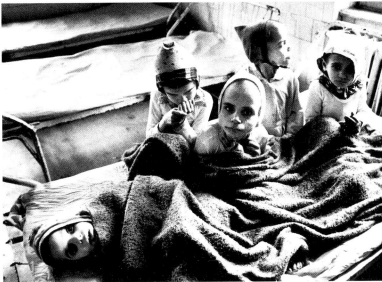

take care of themselves by eating better and getting exercise. People are working to rid the environment of pollution. Filling these needs can prevent disease from starting.

Vaccination Programs

Modern medicine helped rid the world of the disease of smallpox. This was done by vaccinating people throughout the world so they would not get smallpox.

We can rid the world of other diseases also. But vaccination programs cost a lot of money.

Health Care for All
The progress of medicine relies on the research and discoveries made by scientists. It depends also on how much money we are willing to spend for this work. The modern world needs to understand that keeping all the people everywhere in good health will benefit everyone.

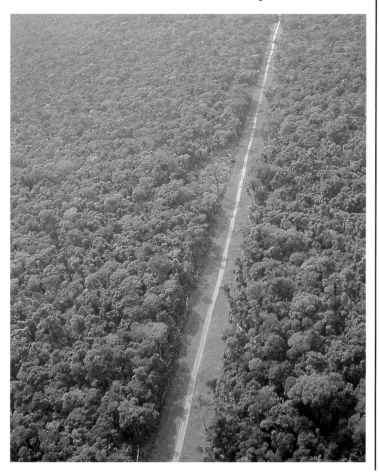

◀ Areas of the Amazon rain forest cut down to make room for a new road. Many of the treatments we use today come from the rain forest. Many more might well be discovered. But they will be lost forever if the rain forest is destroyed.

Glossary

AIDS: These letters stand for a disease called acquired immune deficiency syndrome. AIDS attacks the body's ability to fight infections. Common diseases can become deadly in people who have AIDS.

Anatomy: All the different structures of the body, such as muscles, bones, stomach, kidneys, brain, and the rest. A person who studies anatomy is an anatomist.

Anemia: A blood disease in which there are not enough red blood cells, or the red cells are too small, or the red cells do not have enough hemoglobin — a substance that carries oxygen to all parts of the body. People who have anemia tire out quickly and catch infections easily.

Anesthesia: Numbness, or not feeling anything, in a part of the body, that can result from a drug. A doctor will give a patient an anesthetic drug to keep the person from feeling pain, especially during an operation. A general anesthetic makes a person unconscious.

Antibiotic: A substance, originally from mold, that fights infection by bacteria.

Antiseptic: A chemical substance that kills or disables bacteria, fungi, or viruses.

Artery: A tube that carries blood from the heart to all parts of the body.

Asthma: A disease of the lungs that causes difficulty in breathing from time to time.

Bacteria: One-celled living things that can be seen only under a microscope. Many are harmless, but some cause infections in plants, animals, or humans.

Bacteriology: The study of bacteria. A person who studies bacteria is called a bacteriologist.

Blood vessels: The tubes that carry blood around the inside of a person's body. These tubes are arteries, capillaries, and veins.

Capillary: The tiniest blood vessels. Many can be seen only under a microscope. Capillaries join the arteries and veins.

Cell: The smallest living unit. Some cells can live by themselves, like bacteria. Other living things are made up of many cells.

Cellular pathology: The study of how cells change when they become ill from an infection or other disease.

Chiropractor: A health care professional who treats disease by relieving pressure on nerves and muscles. This pressure can come from bones and joints that are a little out of place.

Chloroform: A gas that can cause anesthesia. It was once used in medicine, but now we have better and safer anesthetics.

Culture: The growth of bacteria in a laboratory dish or bottle where experts can study them. This word also means a group's way of life.

Diabetes: A short name for the disease diabetes mellitus. Diabetes is caused by not having enough of the hormone insulin in the body. This leads to too much sugar in the blood.

Diagnosis: Finding out what a person's illness is. Doctors make a diagnosis by examining the person and asking about any symptoms. They may also need to have laboratory tests done.

Diphtheria: An infection in the throat that can cause a growth that blocks a person's throat and makes it hard to breathe.

Disease: A condition that makes a person sick, or ill. Some diseases result from infections — they are caused by microbes. Other diseases result when something goes wrong in a person's body.

Dispensary: A place where drugs and other medicines are given to patients.

Diviner: A person who uses supranormal means to find water, ores, or the cause of sickness.

Embryology: The study of the growth and development of babies in the mother's womb before they are born.

Fallopian tubes: The tubes through which eggs from female mammals travel to the womb. They are also called oviducts.

Herbalist: A person who uses certain kinds of plants and herbs as medicines to relieve symptoms and cure some illnesses.

Immune: To be safe from catching an infection.

Immunization: Making the body build up protection against a particular disease by giving the person a small amount of disease-causing microbes — bacteria, viruses, or fungi.

Implant: A human-made part that replaces a person's natural part that had to be removed because of disease or damage.

Malaria: A disease caused by a one-celled parasite in a person's red blood cells. The female of a certain kind of mosquito can pass on this disease through a bite. A person with malaria has periods of chills and fever.

Medieval: A word referring to the time in European history from about AD 500-1500.

Mental illness: An illness of the mind that affects a person's behavior, emotions, and reactions to persons and events.

Middle Ages: Another name for the medieval period in European history.

Nobel Prize: One of several prizes in different subjects that are awarded yearly by the Nobel Foundation in Stockholm. Nobel Prizes are given to people who have done something outstanding in their field of work.

Papyrus: A type of writing paper used by ancient Egyptians. Papyrus was made from reeds that grew in the Nile River.

Parasite: Organisms that live on or in other animals or plants, using the larger animal or plant for food and as a home. This can cause illness to the larger animal or plant.

Pathology: The study of what disease does to the body.

Physiology: The study of the way that living things work.

Psychiatry: The branch of medicine that studies and treats mental illnesses.

Radiation: Energy in the form of invisible rays or particles that can damage living tissues. X-rays are one kind of radiation.

Renaissance: A period of European history from the early fourteenth to the late sixteenth centuries. It marks the change from the Middle Ages to the modern age. During this period there was great interest and progress in the arts, literature, and sciences.

Symptoms: The features of an illness that the person with that sickness notices. For example, headaches, other pains, and fever are some symptoms. The pattern of symptoms helps the doctor decide what disease a person may have.

Tissues: A group of cells working together to do a particular job in the body. The entire body is made up of different kinds of tissues.

Transplant: An organ or other human part that replaces a part of a person that has been damaged or diseased. Examples include heart, bone marrow, and kidney transplants.

Tuberculosis: A bacterial infection, mainly of the lungs, causing fever, coughing, and weakened bodily condition. It is also called TB.

Vaccination: Putting into a person's body a weak form of a disease-causing organism so that the body will build up a resistance against that disease. Vaccination is also called inoculation.

Virus: The smallest organism that can live inside plants and animals. It cannot be seen under an ordinary microscope. Some viruses cause disease in plants, animals, and humans.

Index

A **boldface** number shows that the entry is illustrated on that page. The same page often has text about the entry, too.